Portraits

Greyscale Colouring Books
For Adults

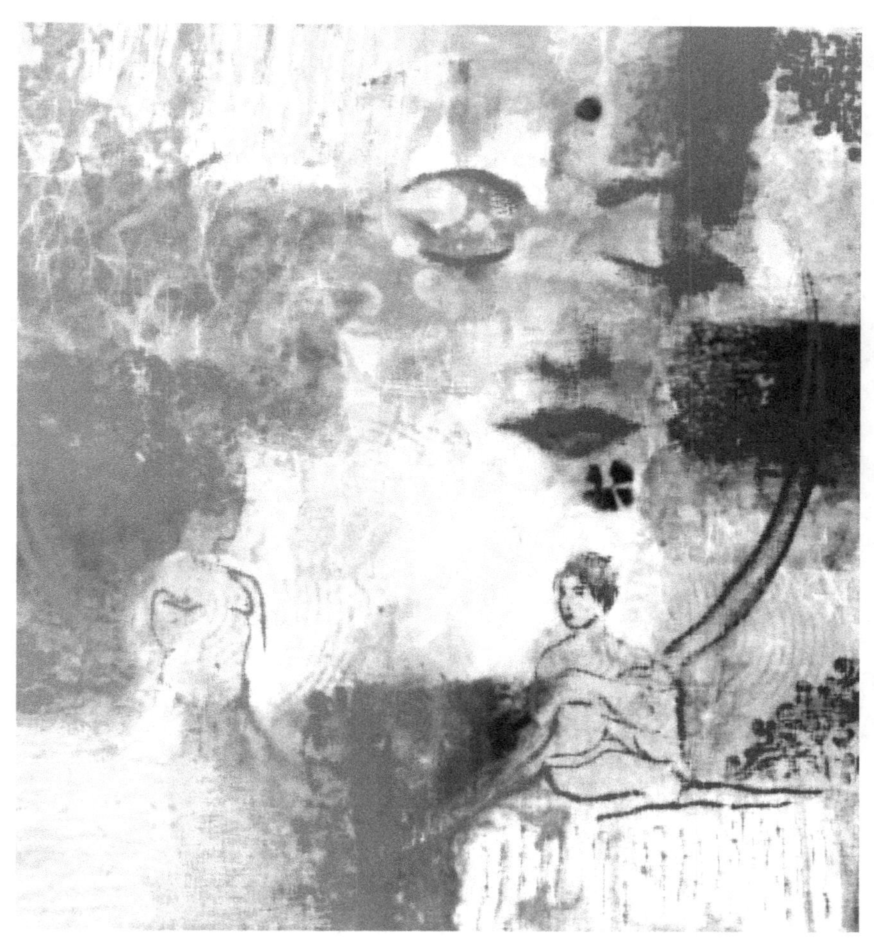

Doris Charest

This book belongs to:

Thinking about the one

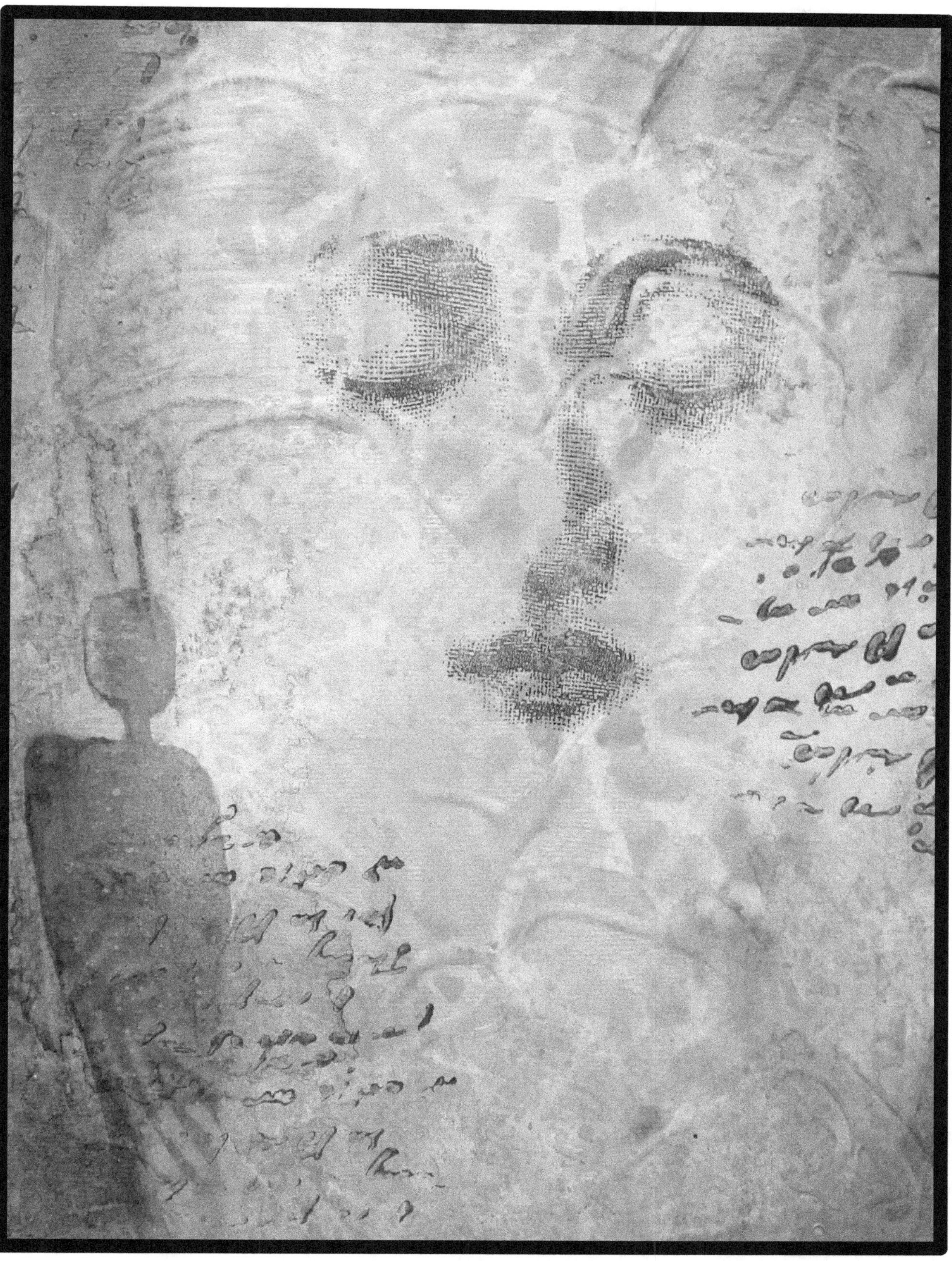

Follow the music

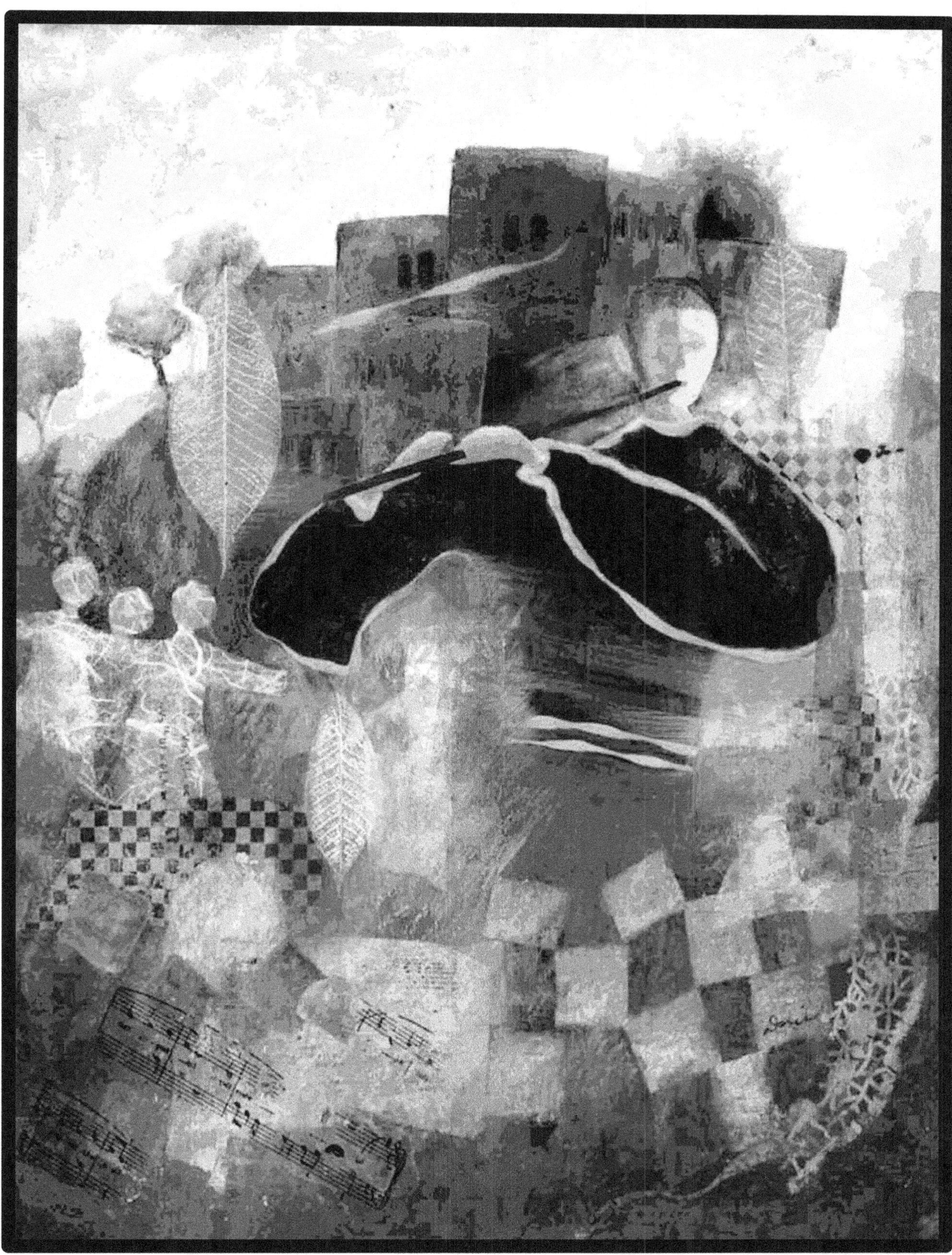

Old times

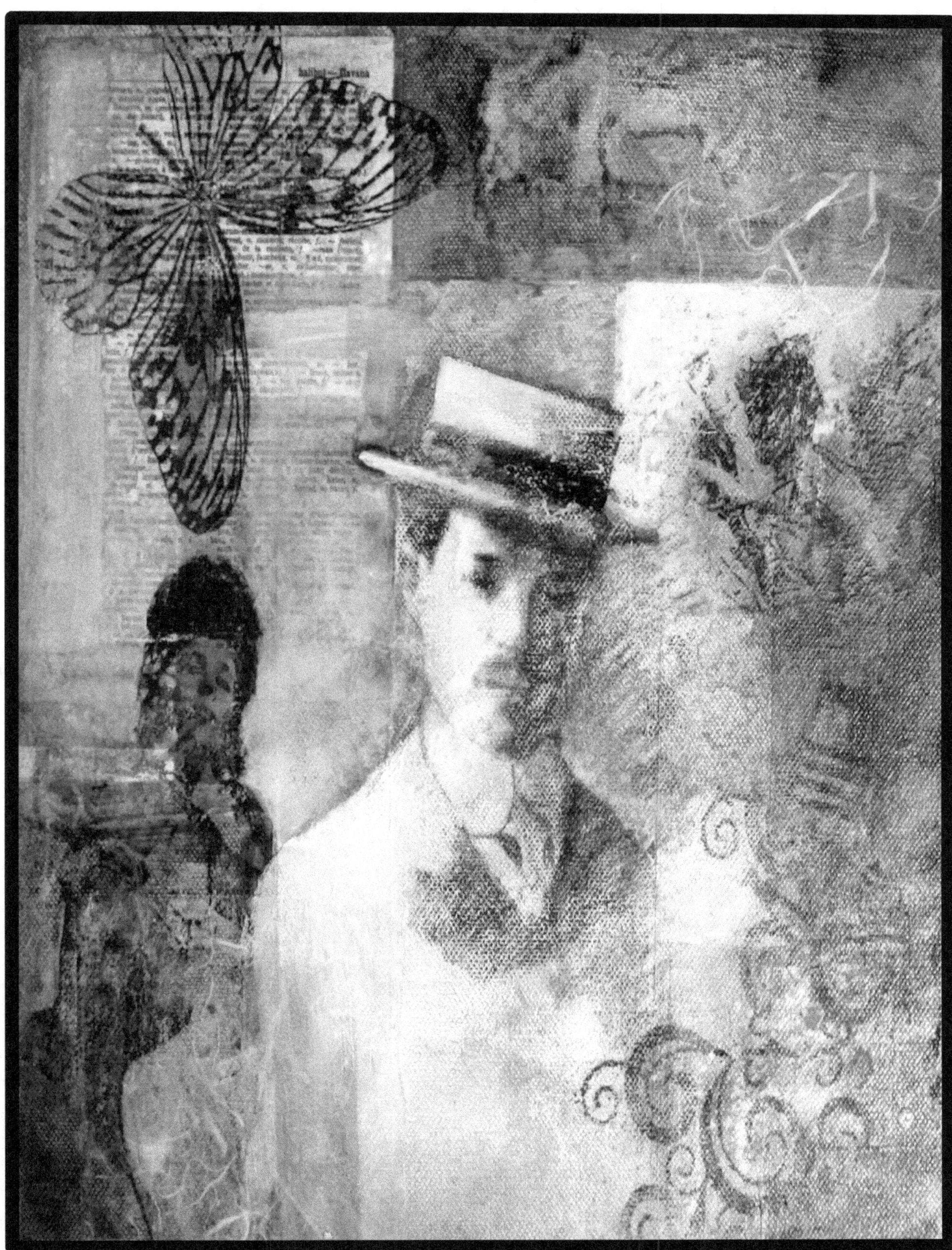

Old times #2

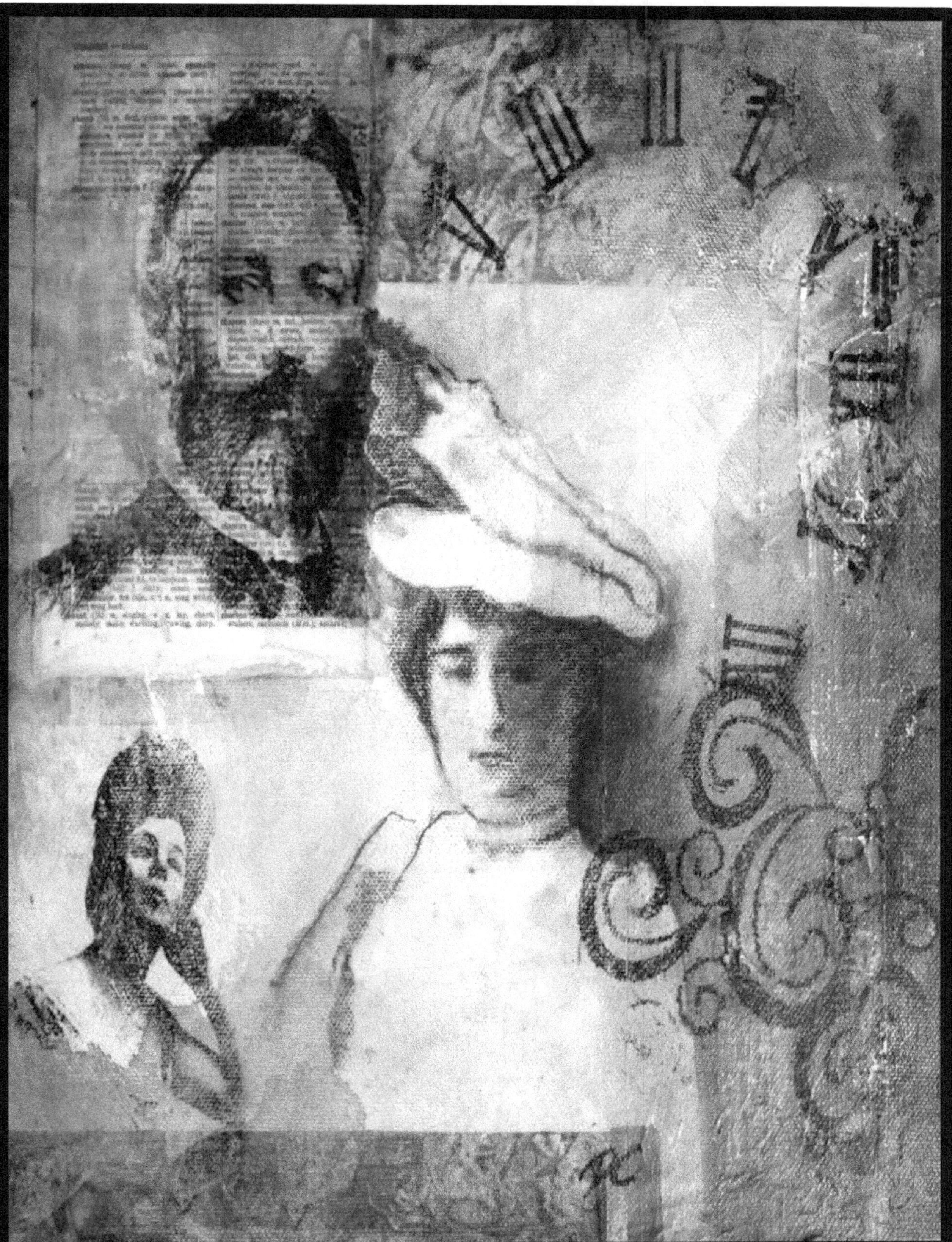

Reach out

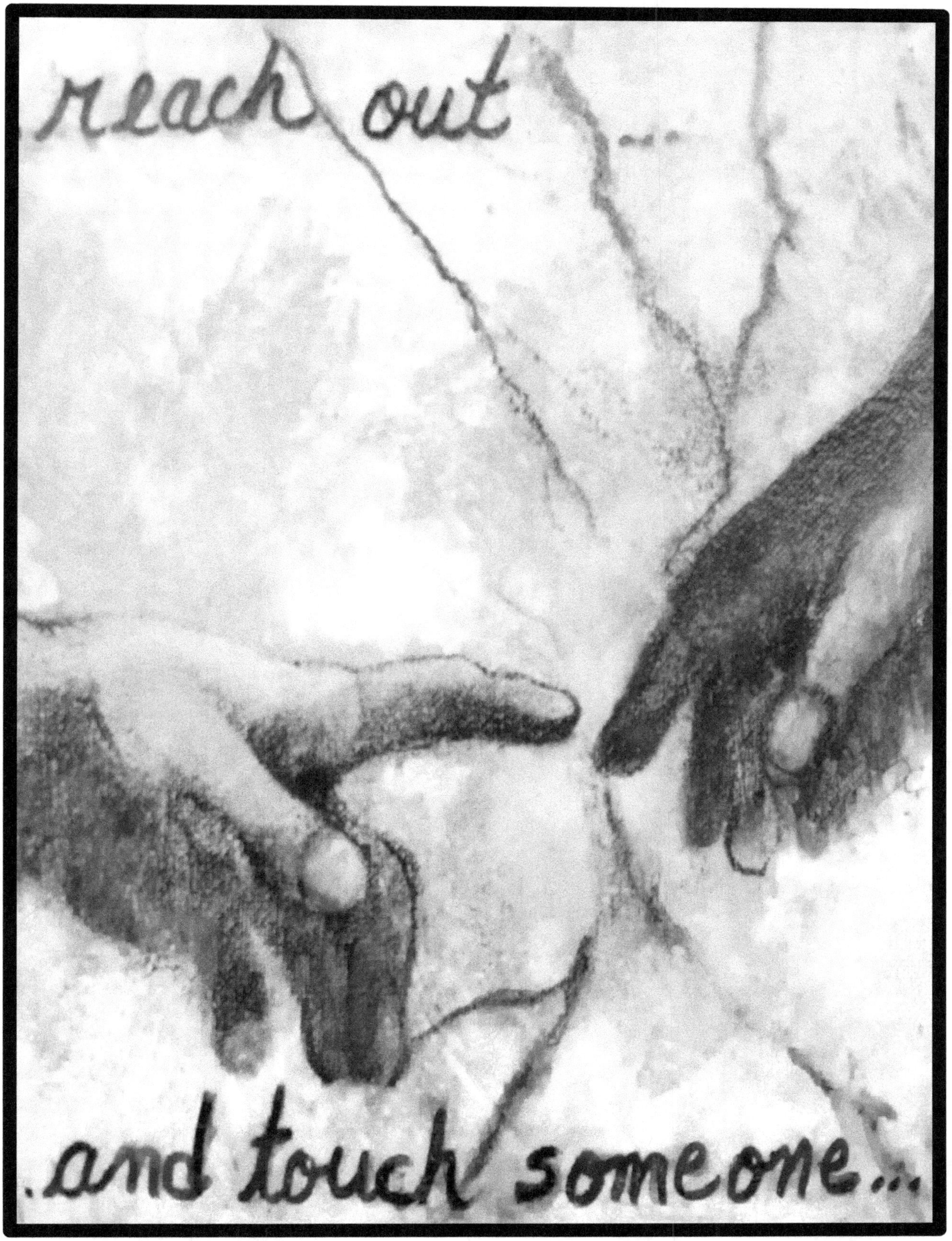

reach out ...
...and touch someone...

Blast out that song

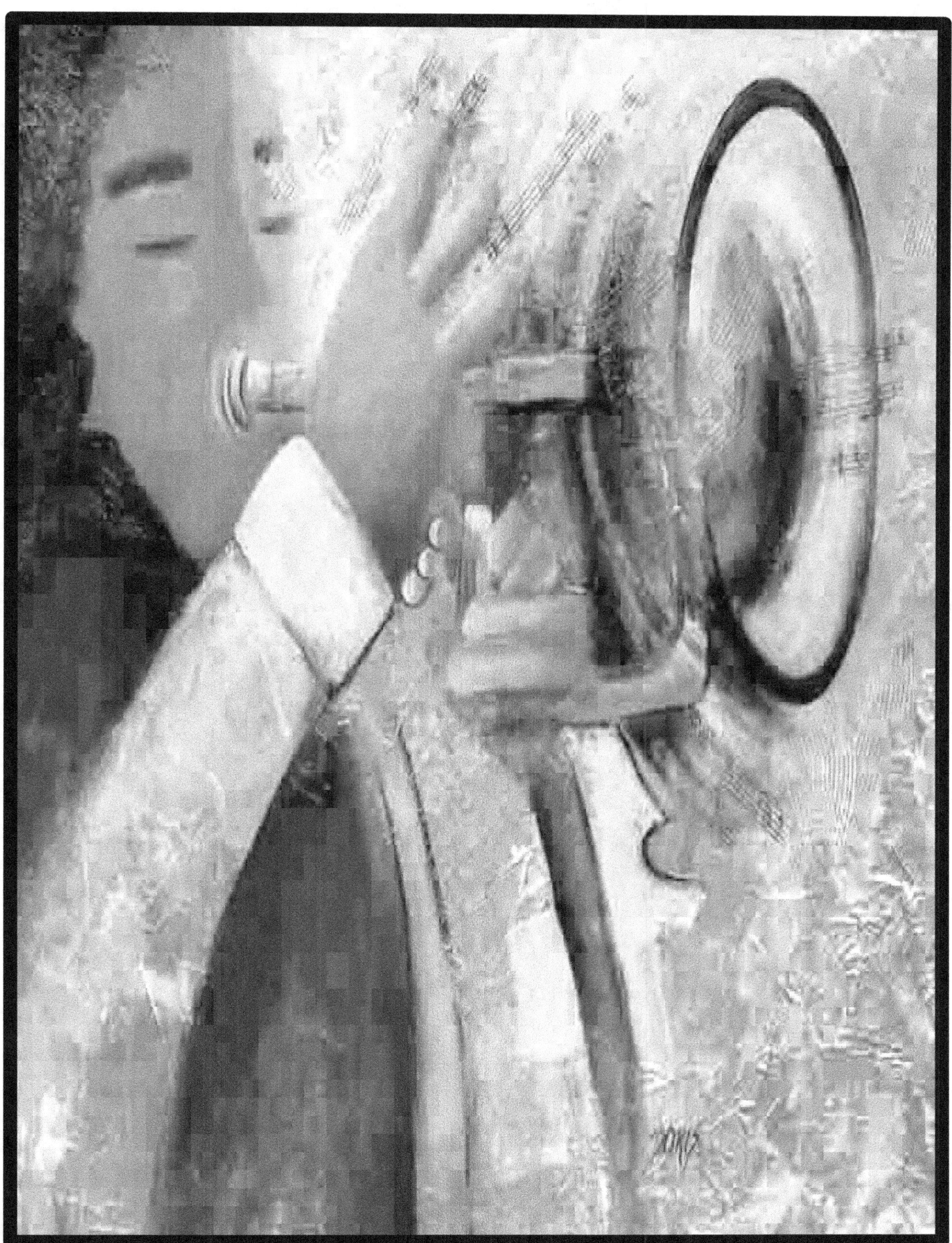

Remembering the good old days

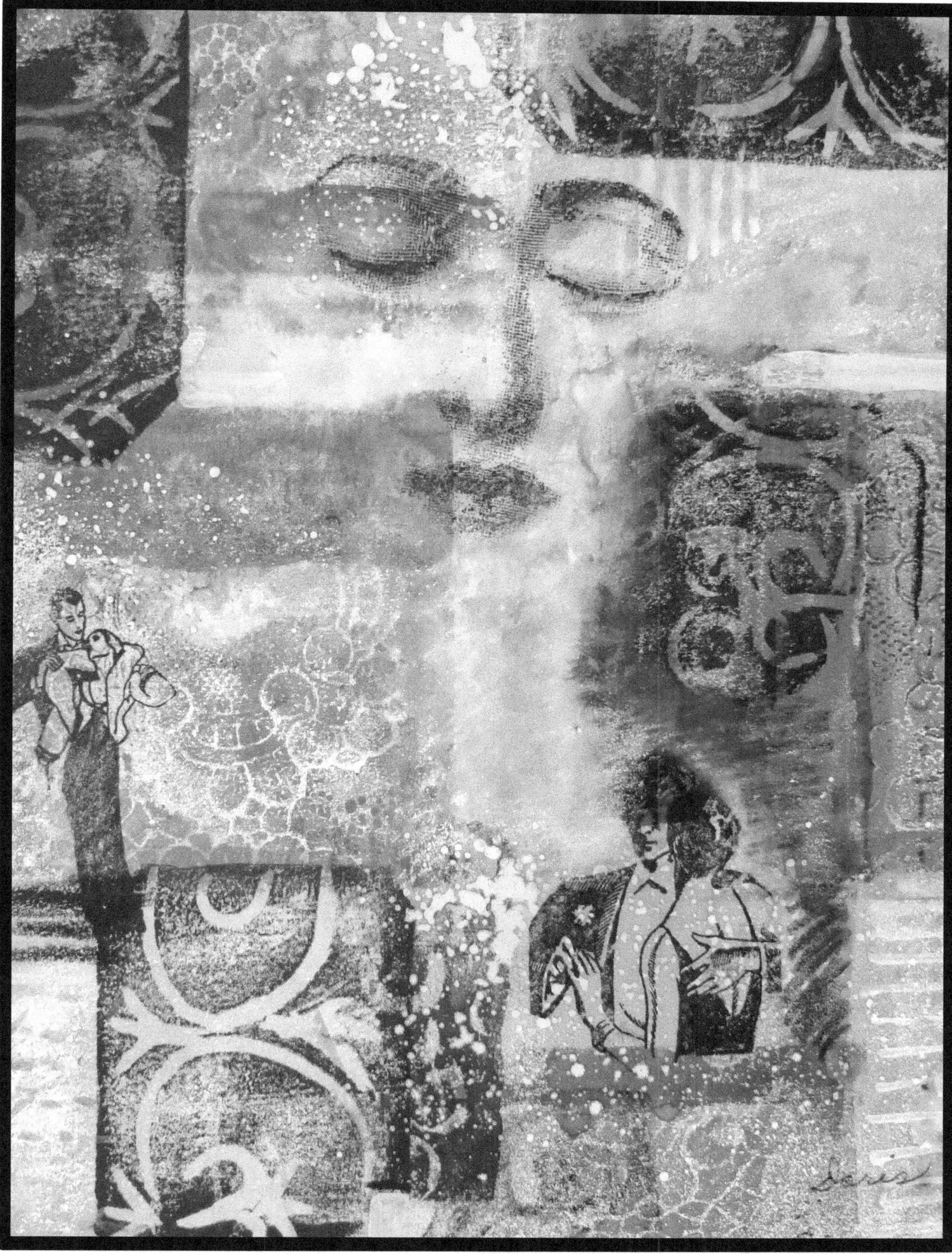

Planning the dance

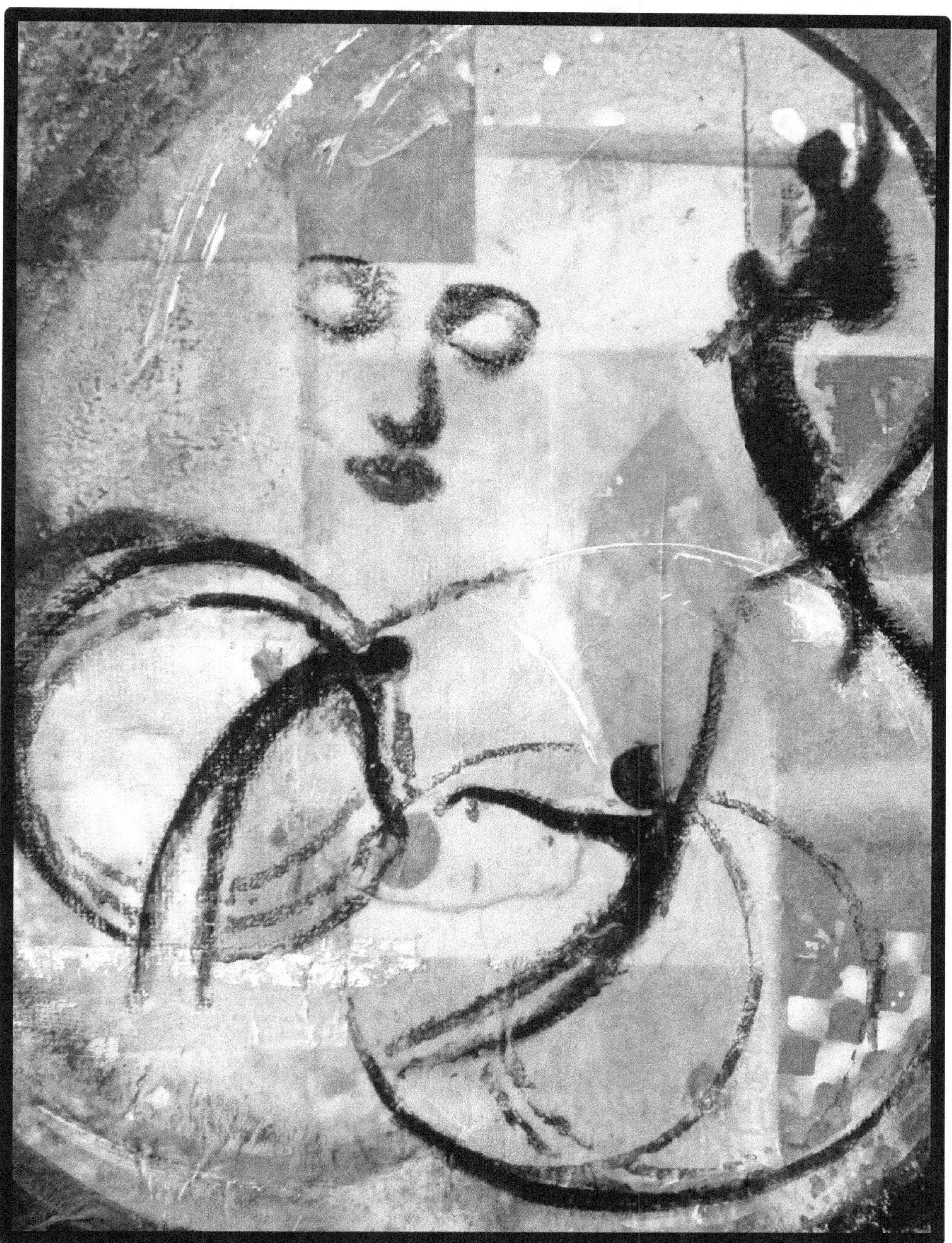

Coming back

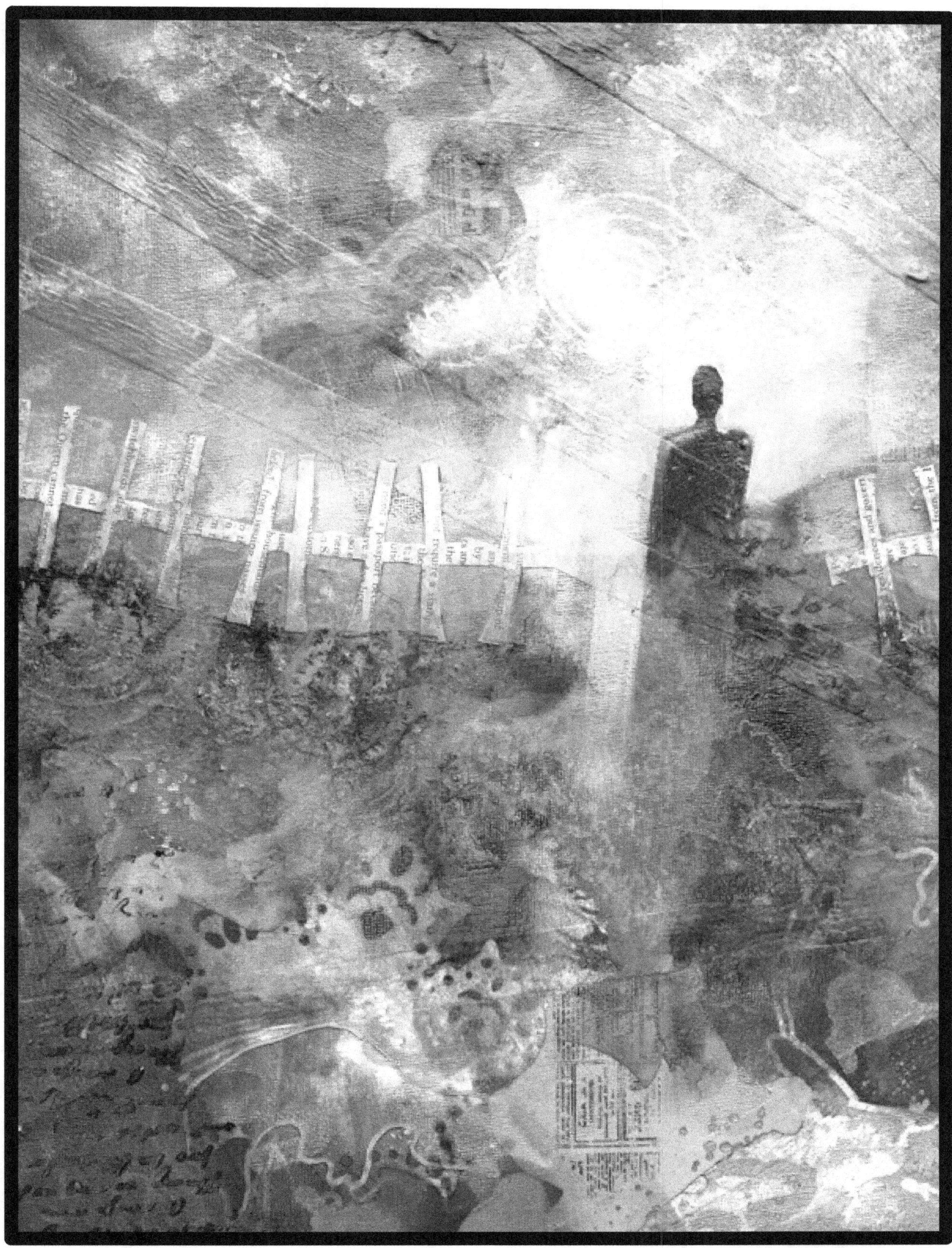

Remembering the 60's

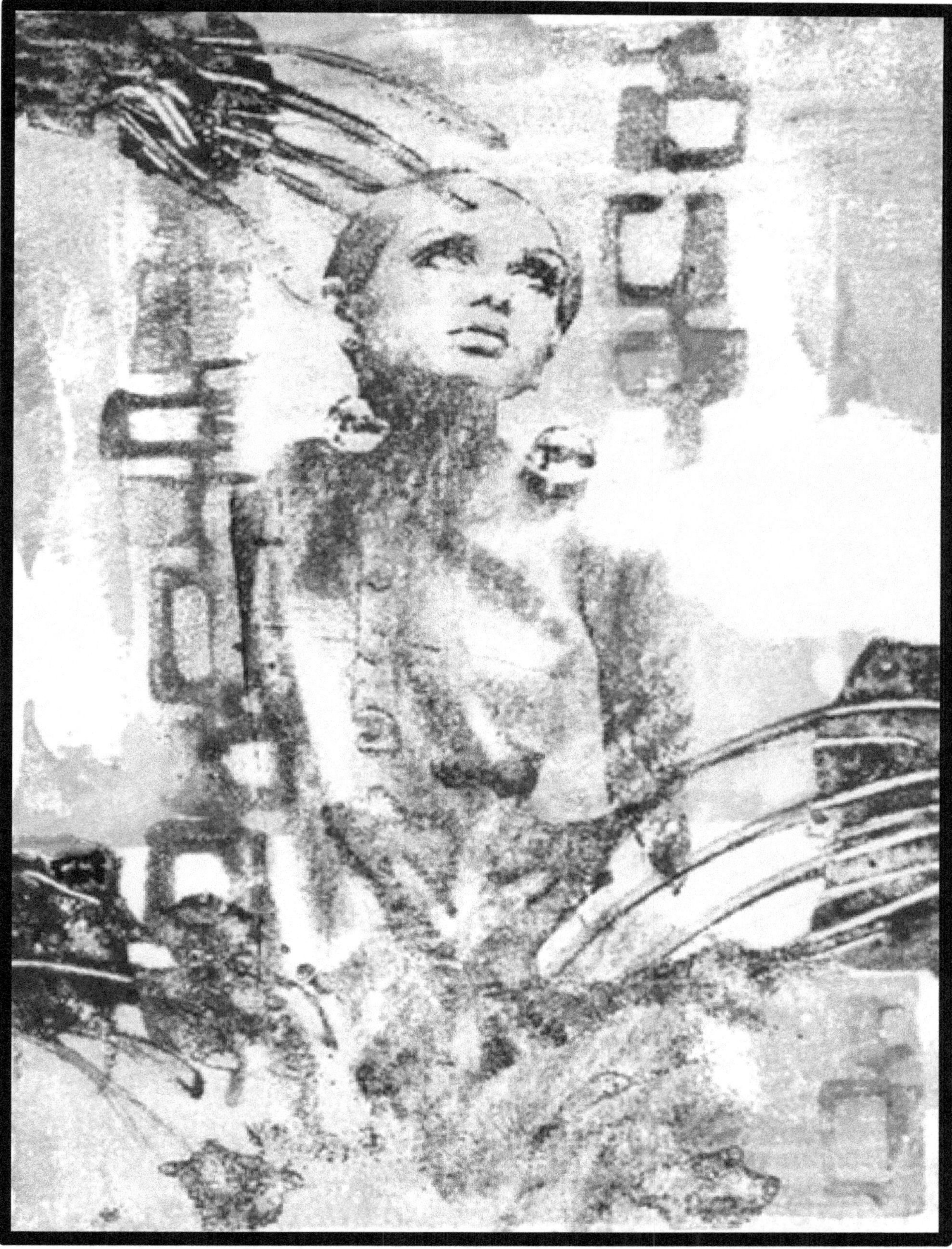

Flamenco dancer

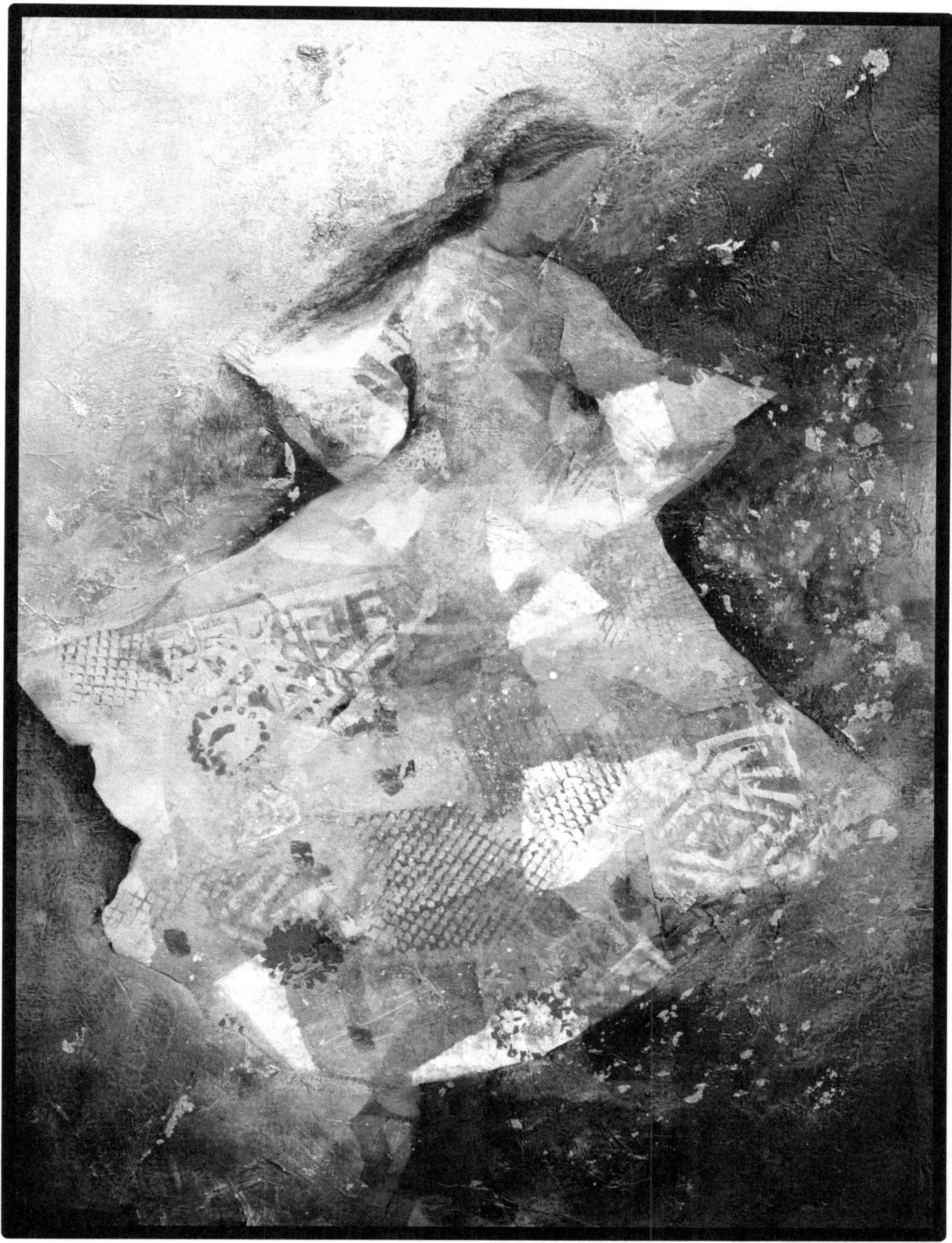

Femme

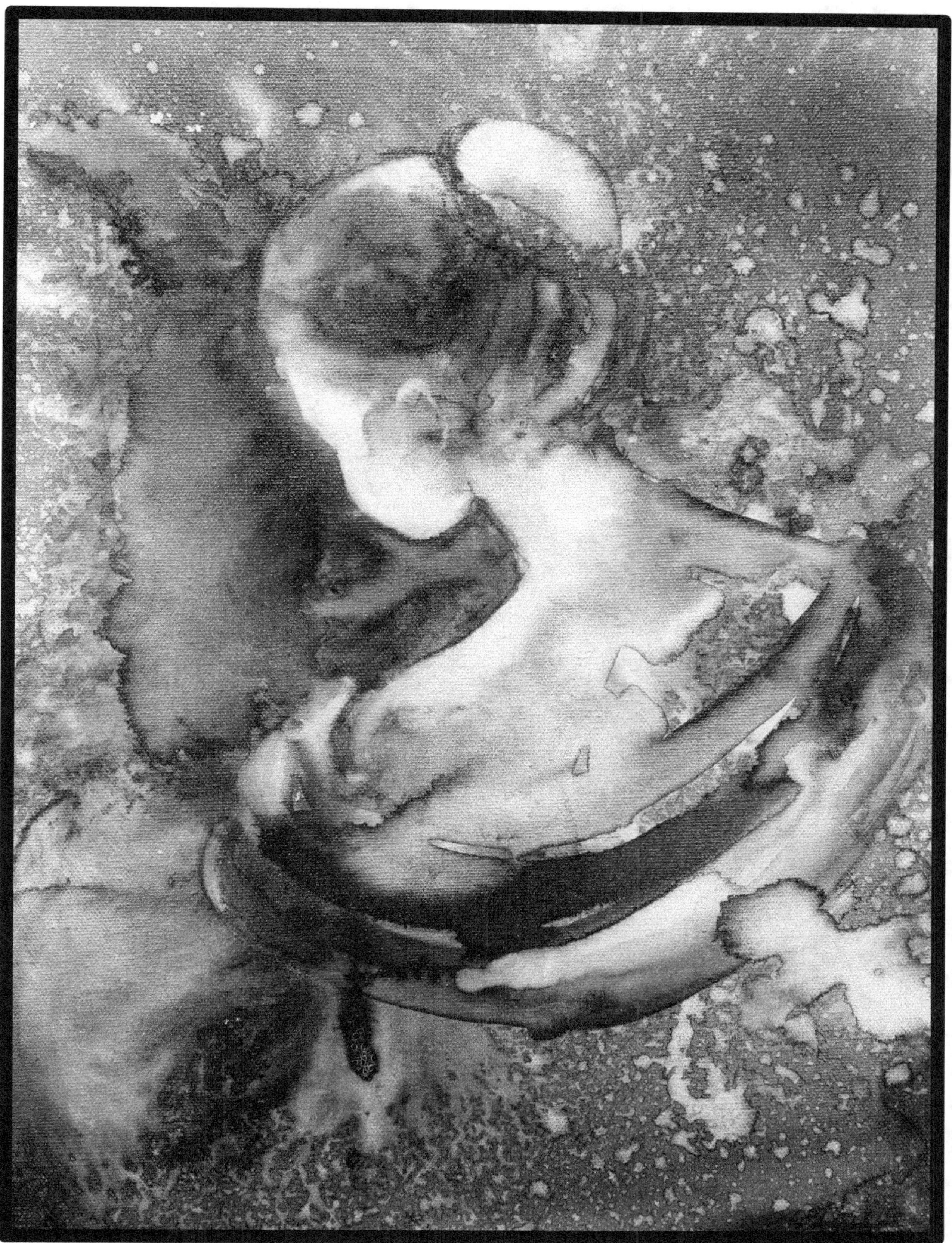

Beauty goddess

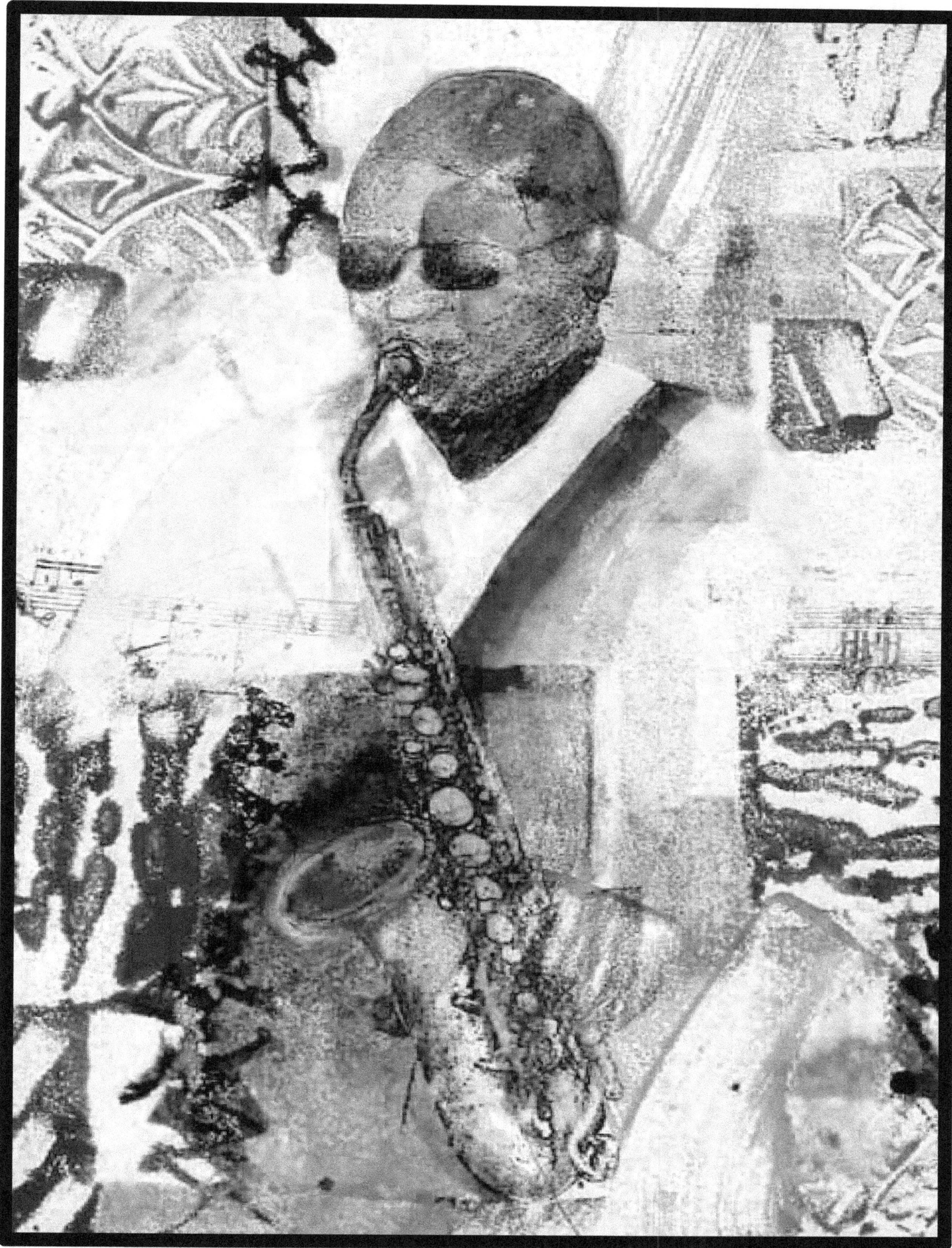

Remembering Marilyn

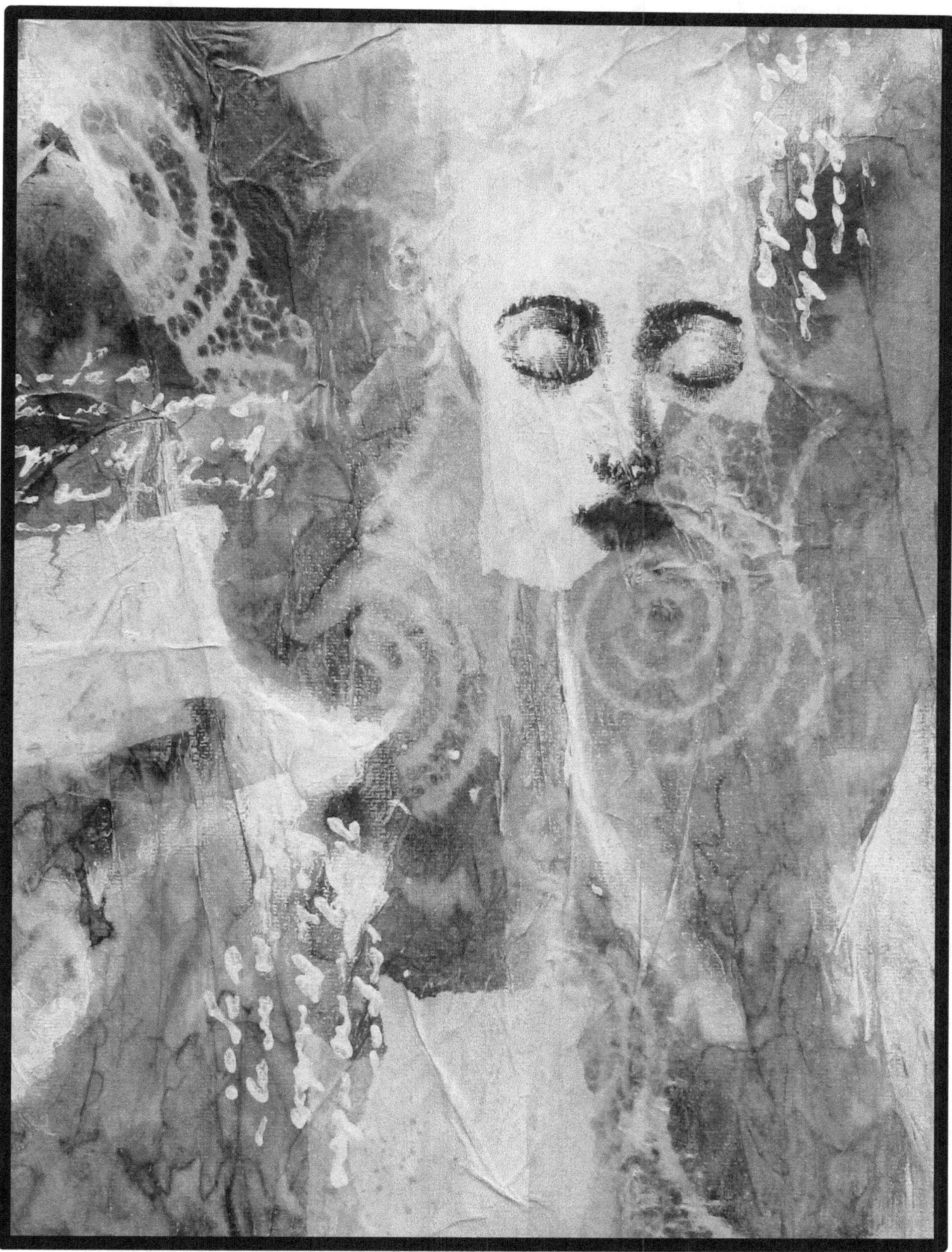

Thinking of her

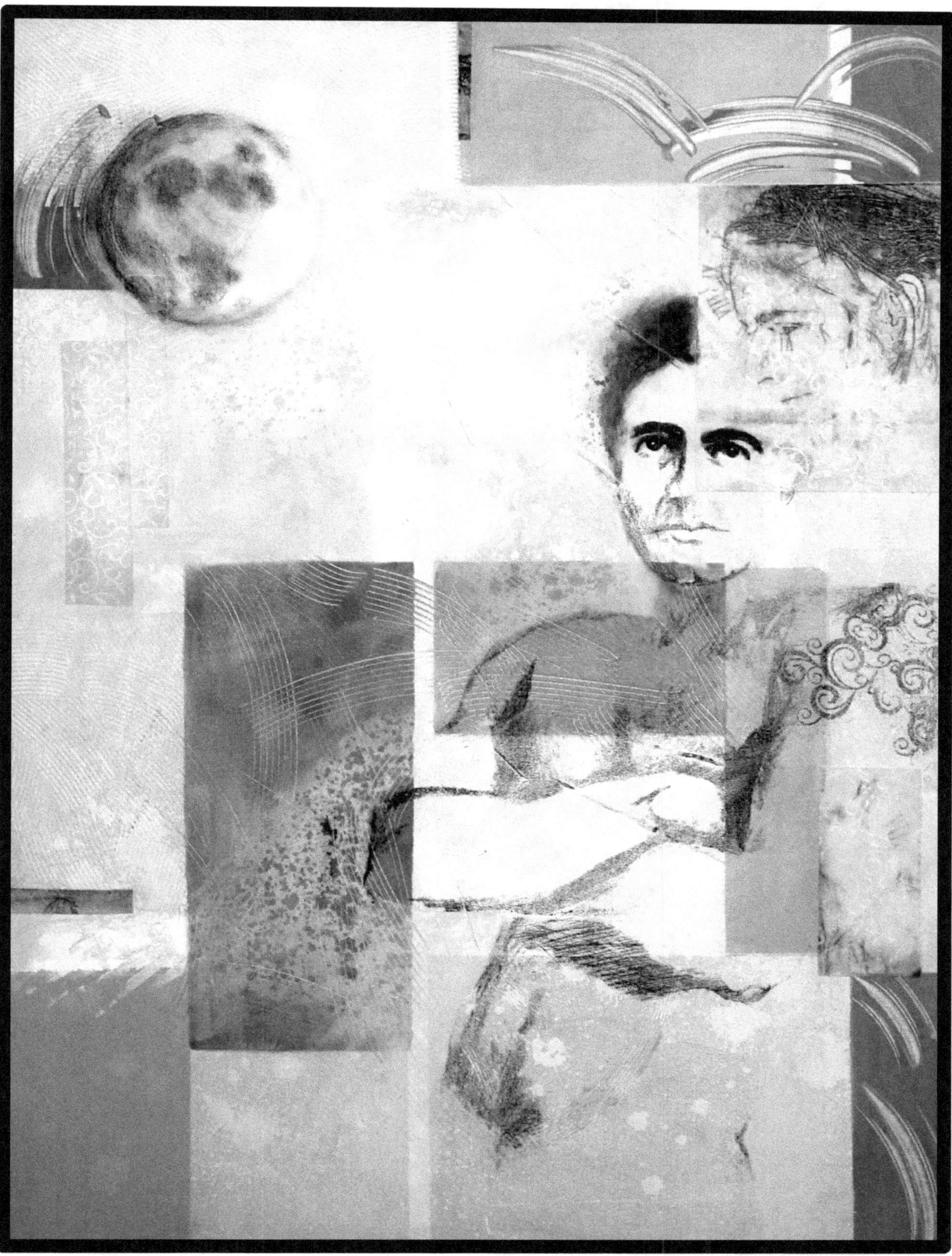

Jamming

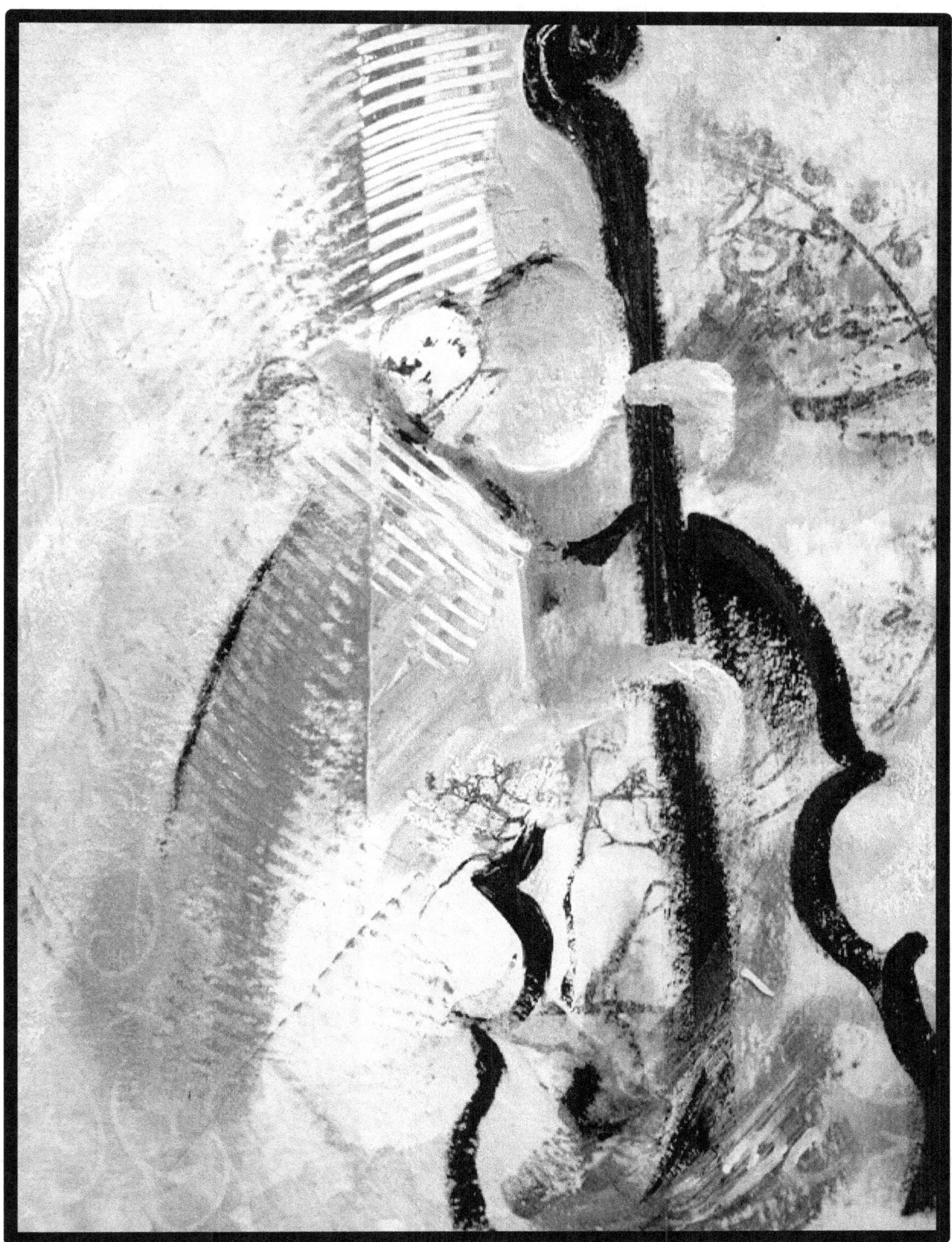

Going to the garden

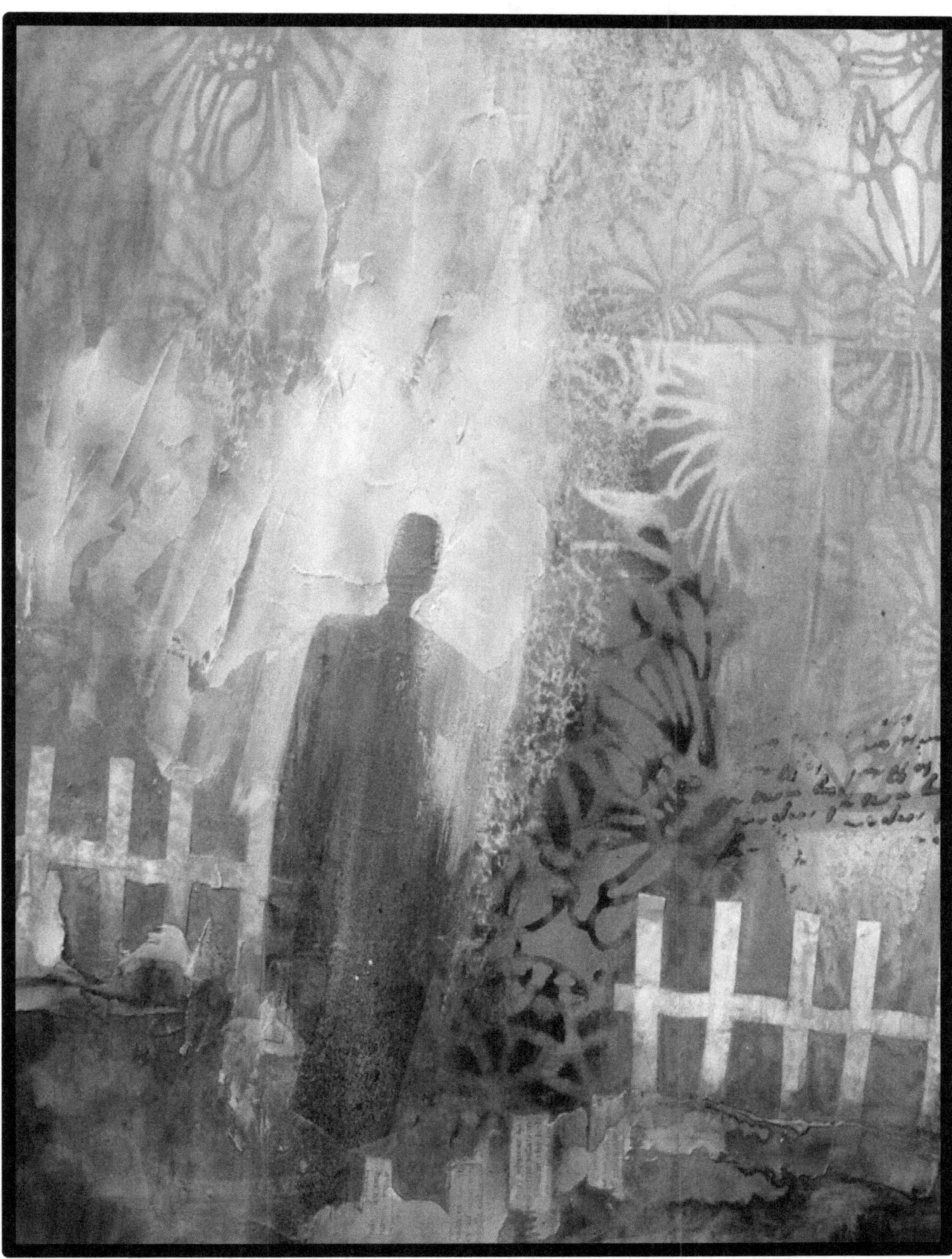

Jazz

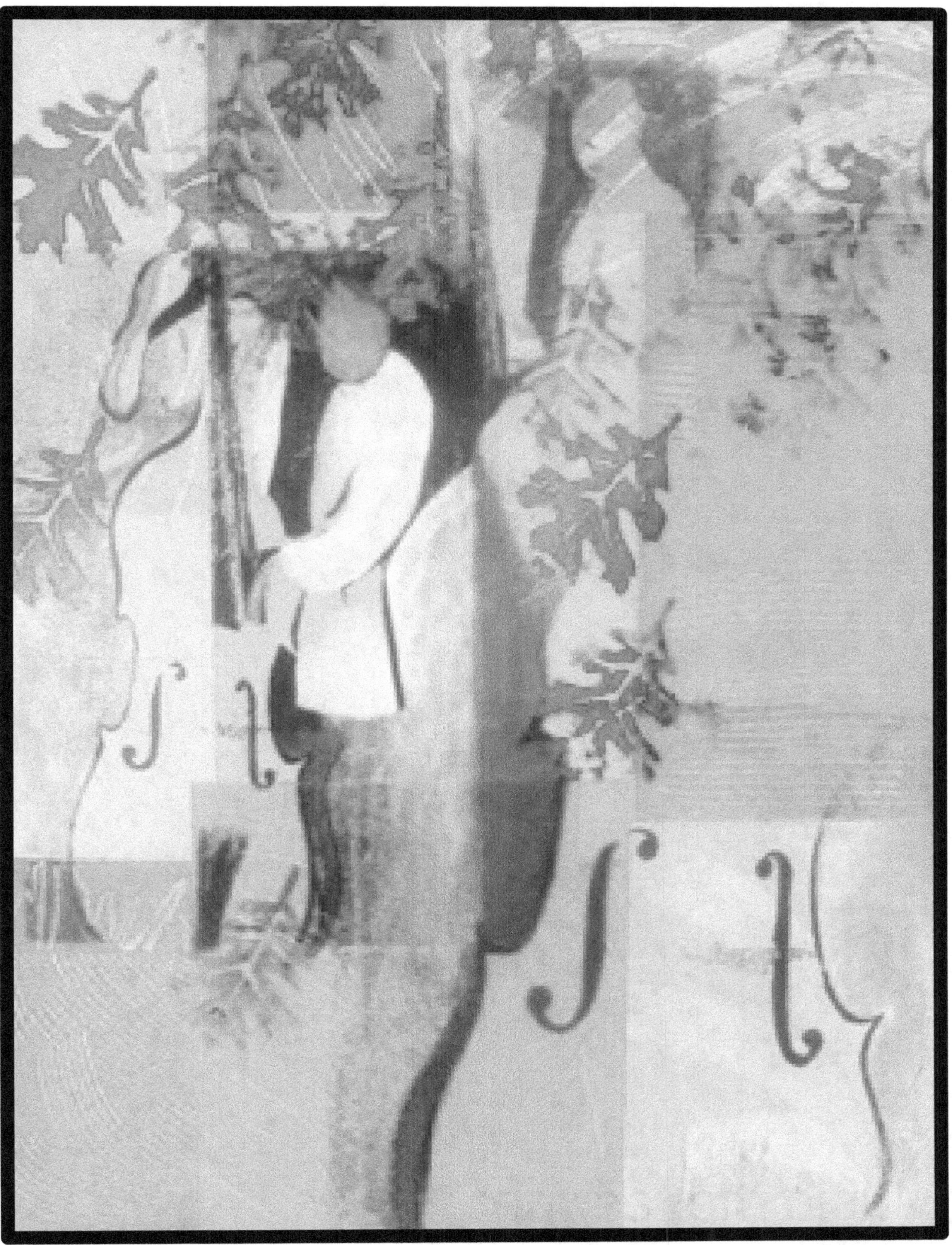

Music moves me

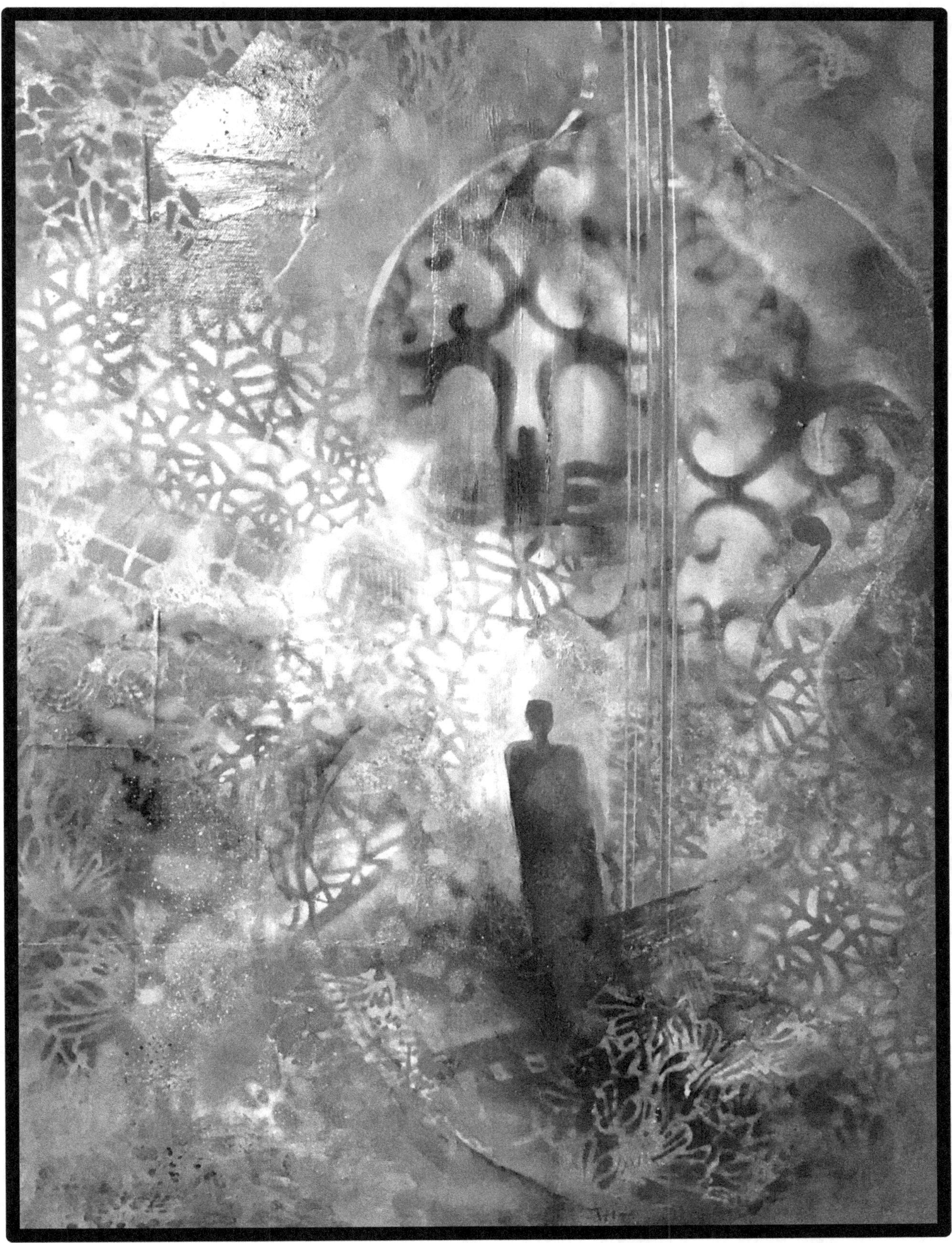

Cuban beat

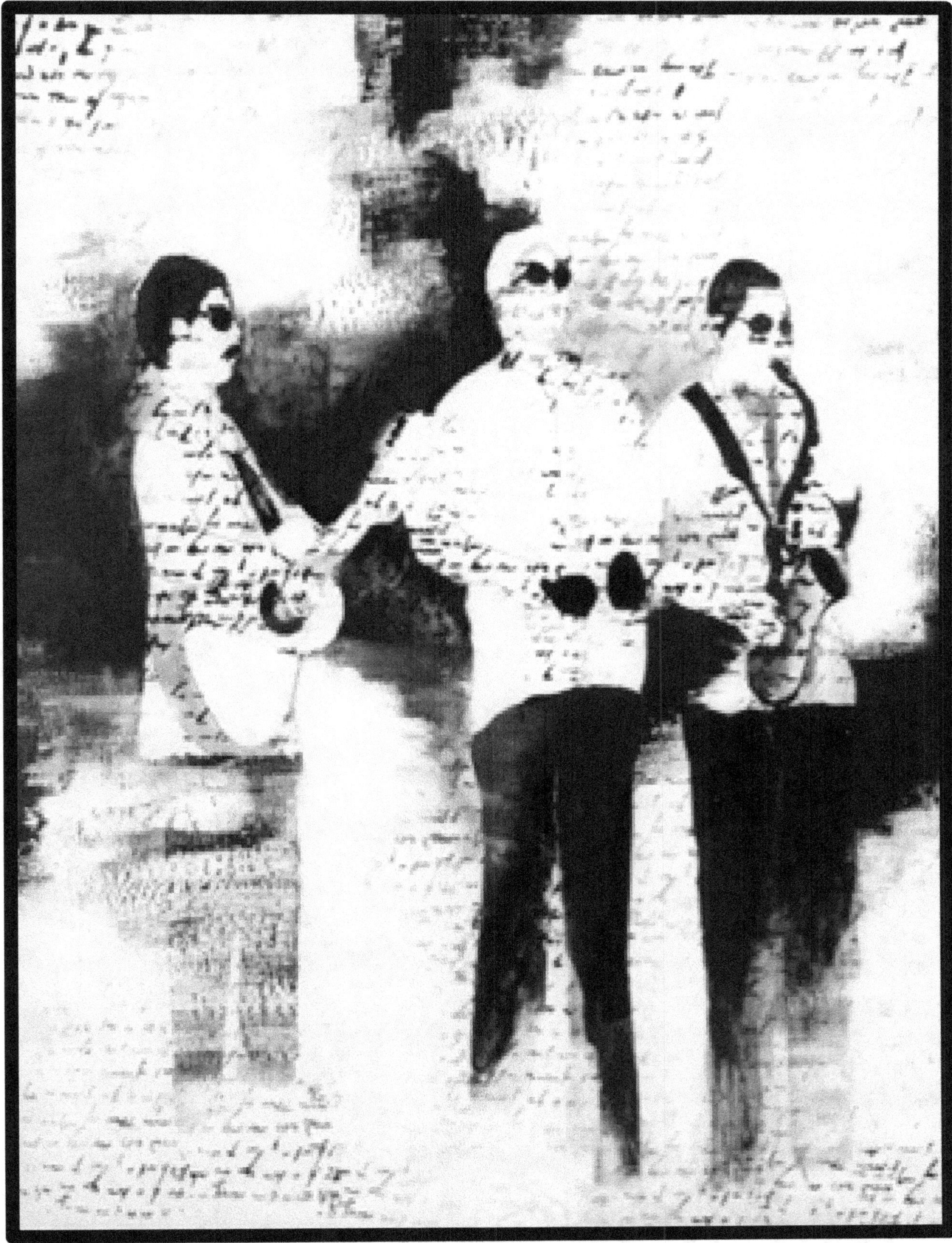

Maze of thoughts

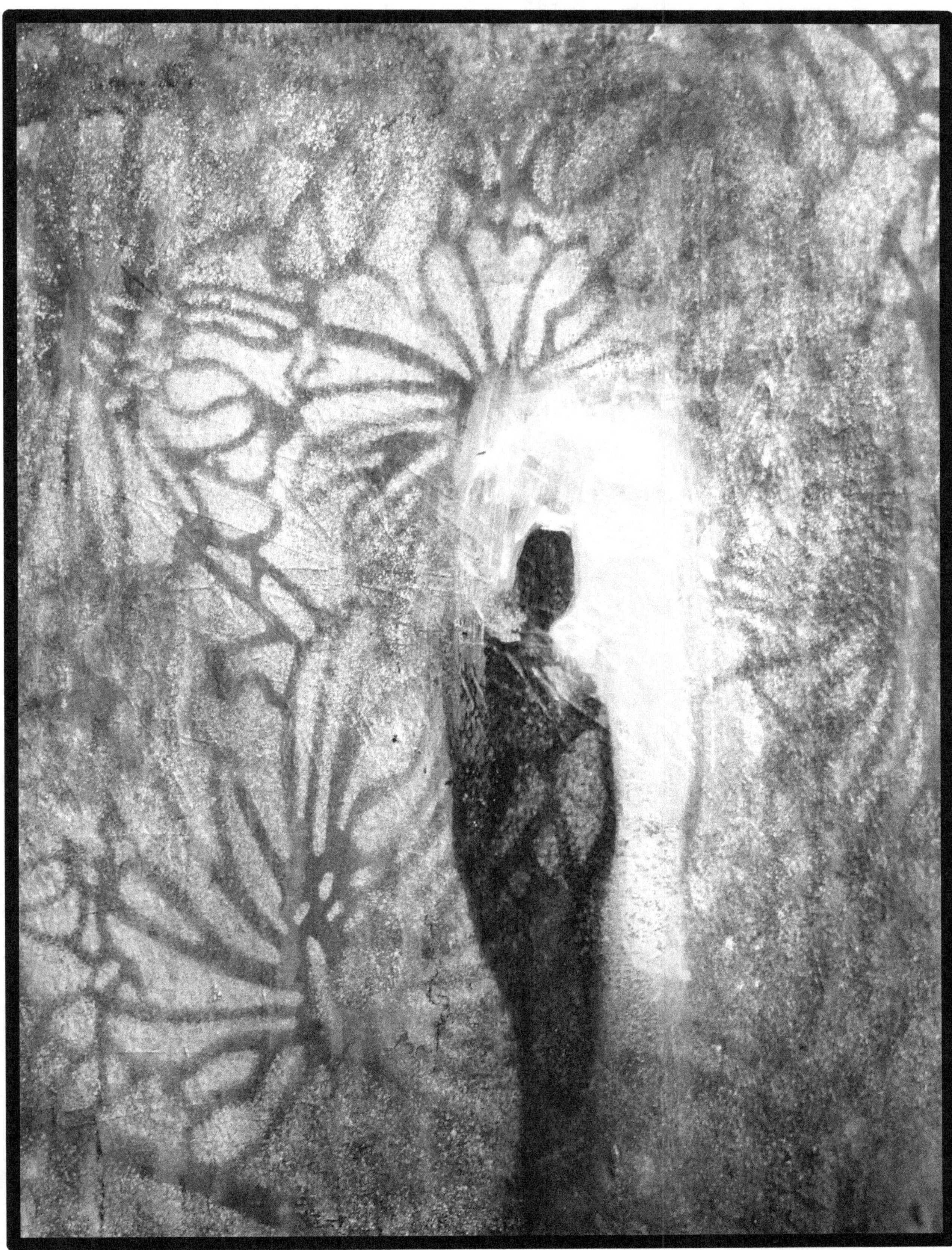

Times past

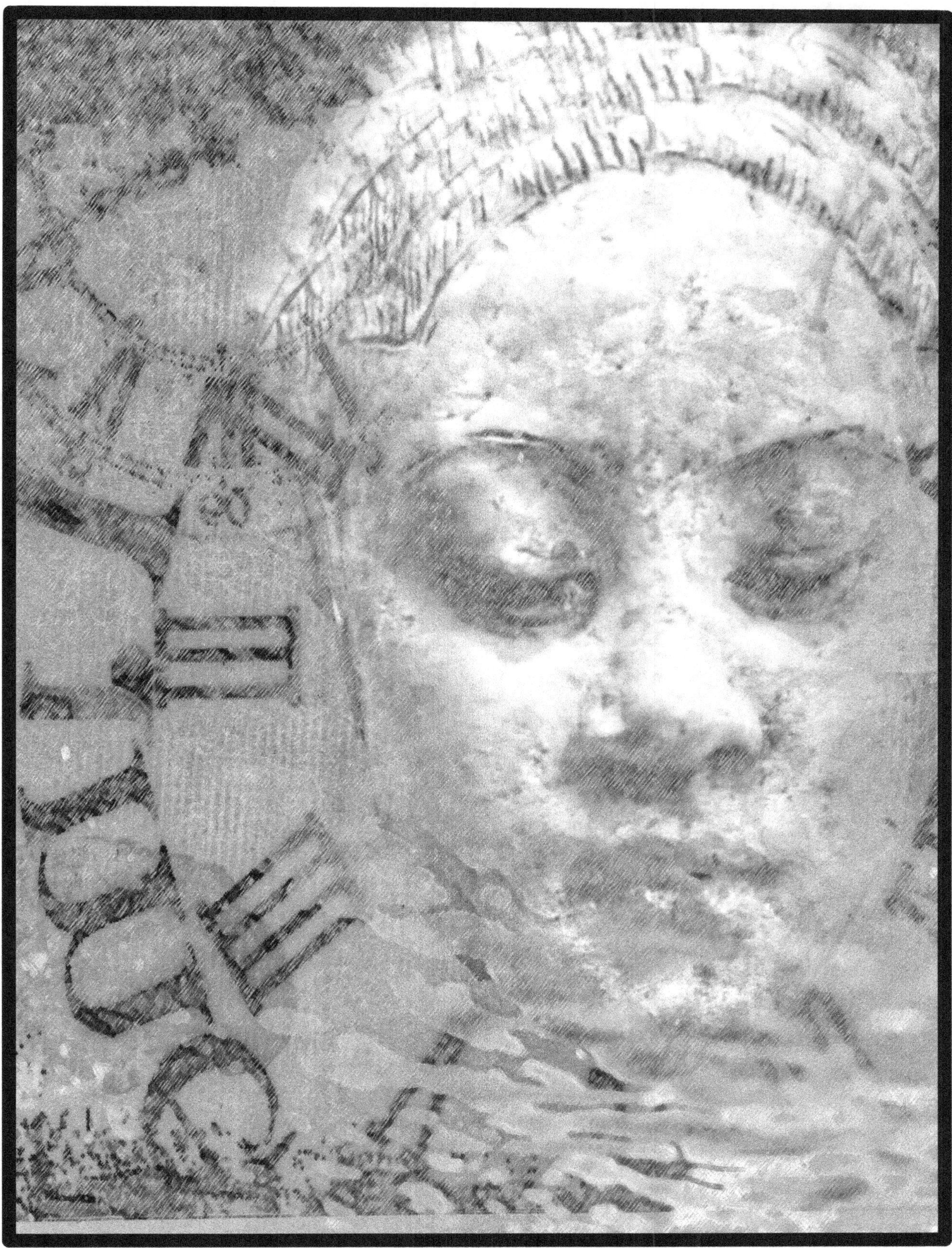

Shy

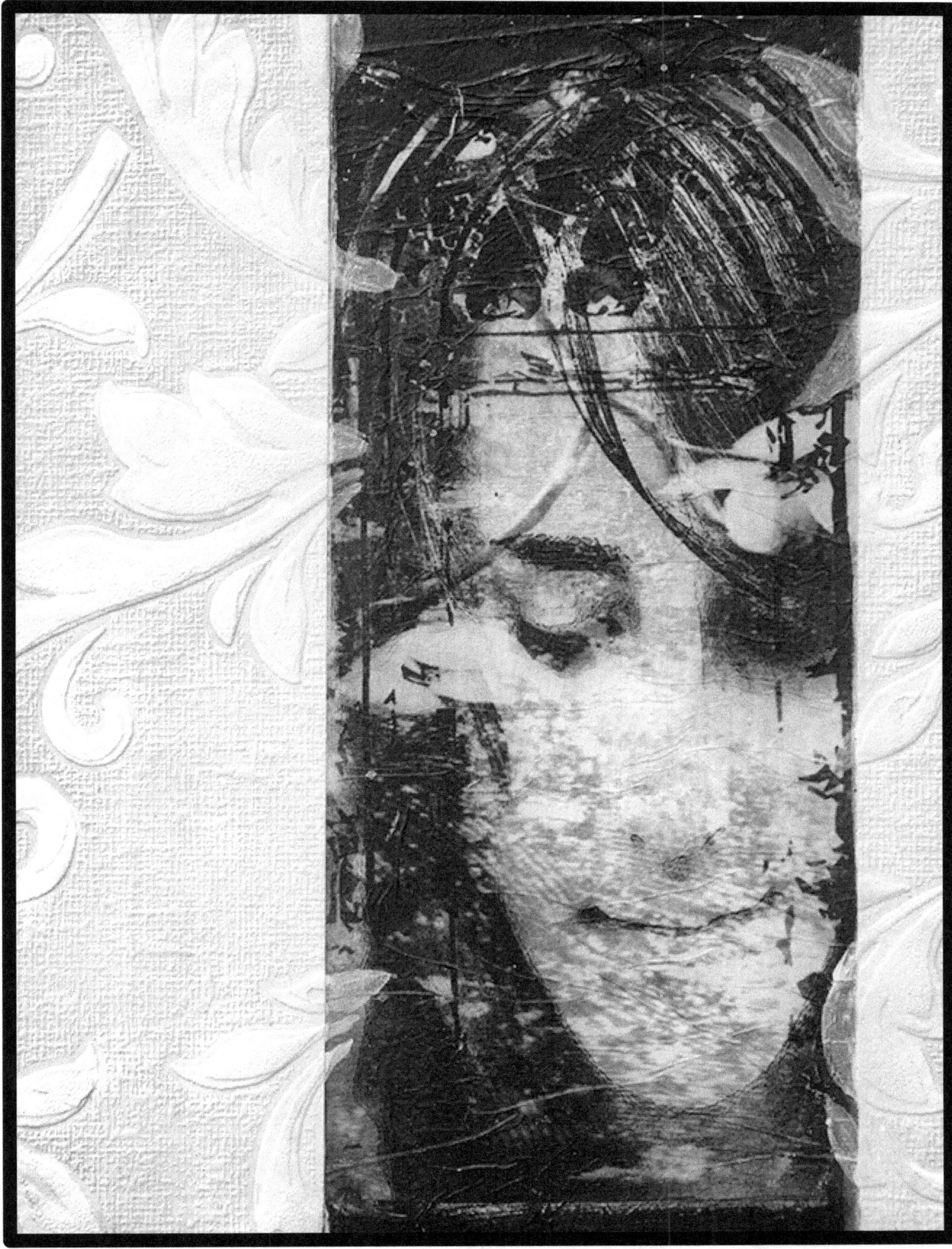

Looking in the mirror

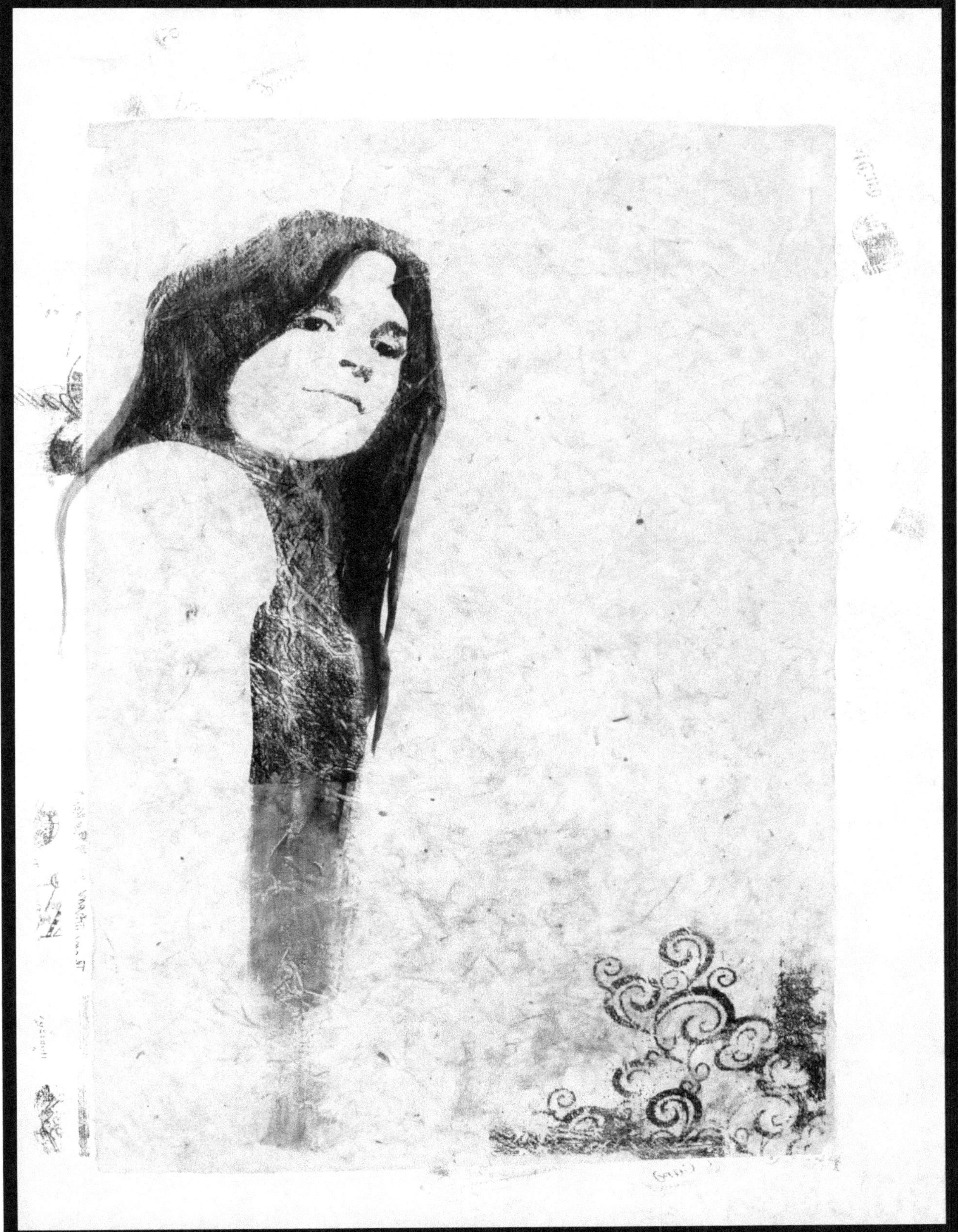

Quiet day

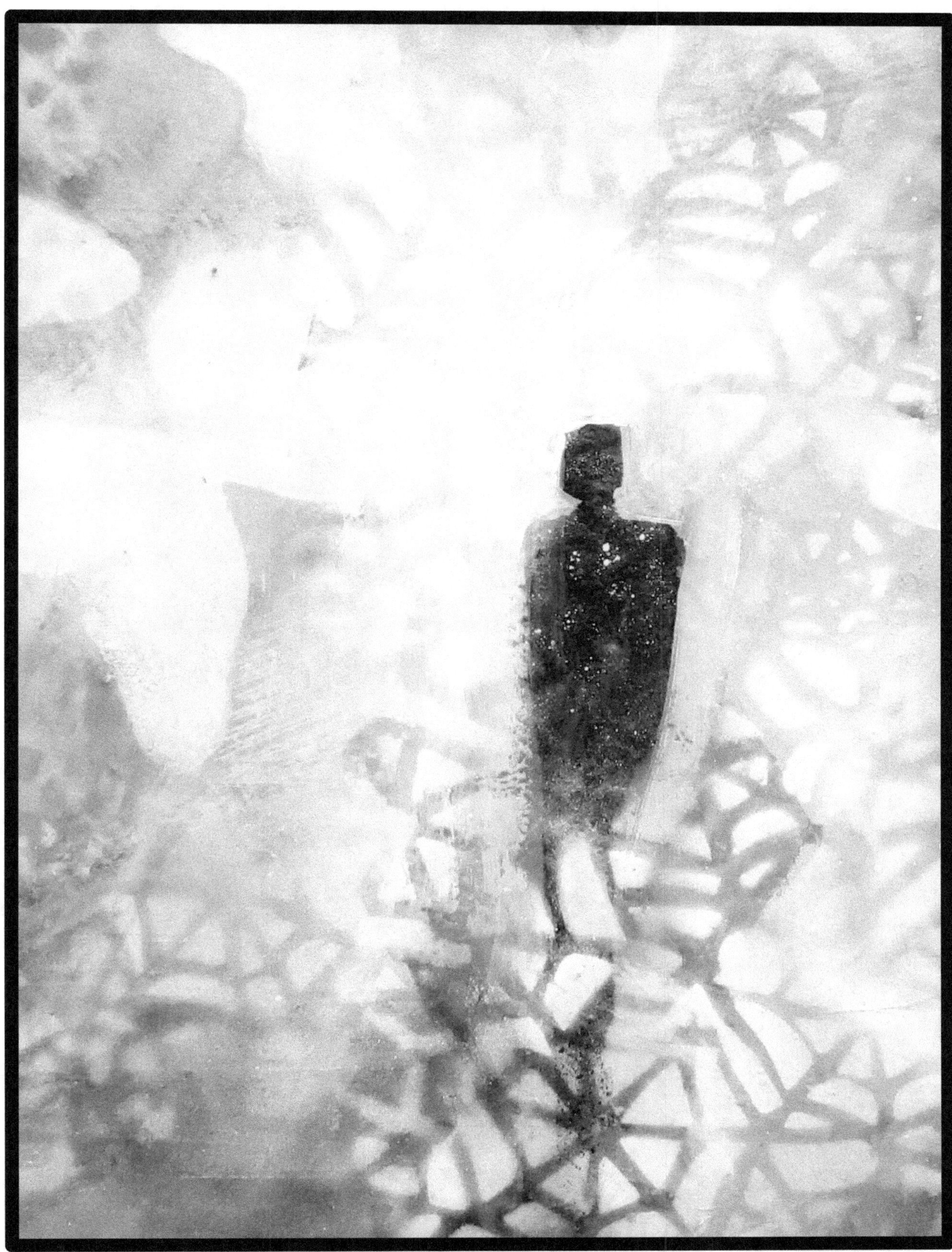

Quiet thoughts

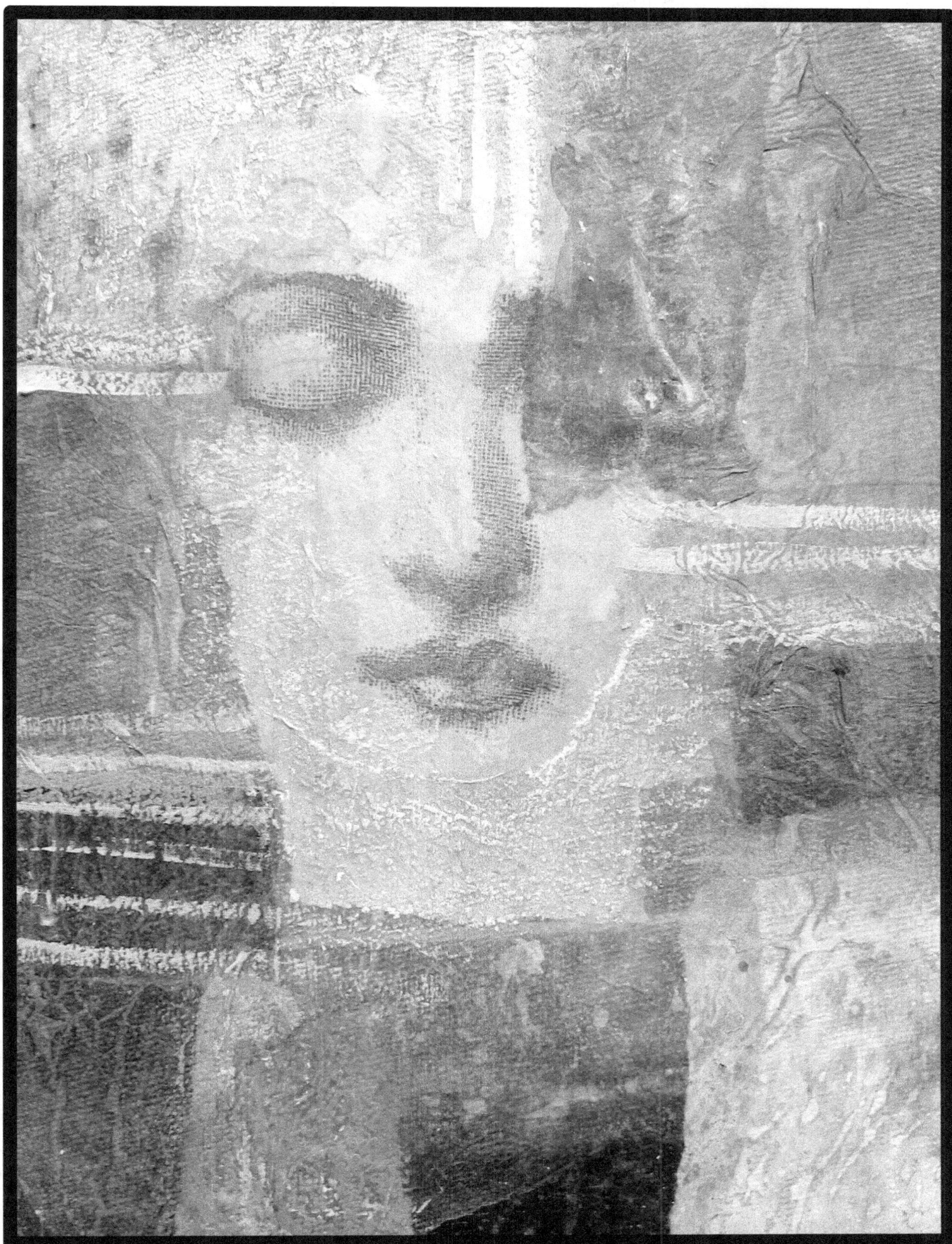